Reversing Catatonia:

The Raw Vegan Plant-Based Detoxification & Regeneration Workbook for Healing Patients.

Volume 8

Health Central

Copyright © 2020

Topics Discussed & Journal Structure

Healing Herbs

Having shared a significant amount of insightful information in the previous volumes, we felt that it would be a good idea to create a volume that is dedicated to sharing knowledge about the different types of herbs that we have had success with. These are herbs that you can also start to incorporate into your protocol today. We trust that these herbs will support your detoxification journey as they have for our patients and ourselves personally.

Herbs are alkalizing and support the healing (and regeneration) process significantly, whilst encouraging you to achieve a deeper detoxification. Always start off with small doses and increase as you see fit. Here are the highly effective herbs that we regularly use with our patients:

Sarsaparilla Root

This herb contains the highest concentration of iron amongst all plants. Providing it is taken alongside the raw diet protocol discussed in previous volumes (predominantly water-dense fruit and some vegetables), it will encourage good health whilst eradicating dis-ease and imbalances that have developed within the body. Iron is the most important mineral amongst other minerals (Chromium, Copper, Iodine, Selenium, Zinc) because just like the others, it is electrical in its form but it also contains a natural magnetism and this magnetism is crucial for good health and life to co-exist.

Burdock Root

Burdock Root has been used for hundreds of years for its medicinal properties. It was traditionally used as a blood purifier. It can be taken alone or with other herbs (such as Yellow Dock and Sarsaparilla). This herb increases the blood circulation to the skin and this subsequently supports the process of detoxification via the epidermal tissue/skin through perspiration. The skin is our largest eliminative organ and so it is important that we focus on this area during our detoxification and healing phase.

Burdock Root has also been found to remove bacteria and fungus cultures from within our digestive tract and this in-turn reduces cooked food cravings. Additionally it is a diuretic which means that it will encourage the kidneys to filter out impurities from the lymphatic system (the body's main sewage system that cleanses everything from the blood to tissue/cells). With any type of diuretic, be sure to keep up water intake and stay hydrated.

Yellow Dock Root

Yellow dock root is another well-proven detoxifying herb which stimulates the upper and lower digestive tract. You will find that it will support bowel movements for the elimination of any aged/lingering waste that may be present within the intestines. There is also the added benefit of increased toxin elimination through improved kidney filtration. It is important to maintain an efficient rate of waste elimination as this will reduce the accumulation and congestion of toxins within your lymphatic system, tissue and bloodstream.

Dandelion Herb

Boasting a series of detoxification benefits (increased bowel movement and urination frequency), dandelions are also rich in calcium, which is essential for the growth and strength of your bones. Comprising of antioxidants such as Vitamin C and Luteolin, this herb will also support your liver which is one of the most important organs in your body.

German Chamomile

Very good for upper body and brain circulation, German Chamomile calms the central nervous system as it gets to work.

It will help with balancing out your digestive system which must be in good order as it plays a crucial role in healing.

Elder Berry

This is a great herb for boosting the immune system and reducing any immediate pain that is being experienced. It will support detoxification through the opening of your bowels and kidneys – including your skin (the 3rd kidney) through increased perspiration/sweating out of toxins.

Organic Kelp/Bladderwrack

Bladderwrack is a form of kelp that has been used medicinally for centuries. It is very high in Iodine and this stimulates healthy thyroid function/metabolism along with improved upper blood circulation, whilst lowering internal and external inflammation. Packed with a wide variety of minerals, Bladderwrack will support the passage of toxins out of your body through your skin/pores whilst nourishing your cells and reducing any excessive fluid retention.

Sea Moss/Irish Moss

This is a powerful Superfood which is extremely nourishing for the cells. It will supply your body with nutrition on a deep cellular level – all whilst removing the dis-ease causing acids and mucus from your body. We have found it to also offer great strength to bones and connective tissue.

Red Clover

Red Clover is a powerful internal cleanser and healer which supports the kidneys and gut with improved toxin disposal and filtration out of the body. It is very good for upper body blood circulation, throughout the organs – including the skin. This increased flow of blood comes with multiple healing, preventative and pain relief benefits.

Red Raspberry Leaf

As its name suggests, Red Raspberry Leaf is the leaf of the red raspberry plant. It is well known for its beneficial nature for females at all stages of their lives. It is naturally high in Magnesium, Potassium, Iron and B-Vitamins – and can therefore help overcome nausea, cramps, and improve sleep quality. Additionally, it has great benefits for the female reproductive system as it has been known to strengthen the uterus and pelvic muscles.

Stinging Nettle Leaf

This herb dates back to the ancient Greek era. It is effective as a diuretic (opening up the kidneys) and laxative (for increased bowel movement) – both playing vital roles during detoxification. We use this herb regularly, as a blood purifier, for a variety of conditions – ranging from cancers to diabetes. Nettle leaf is amongst the most valuable herbal remedies available with great healing and astringent (suction) qualities.

Milk Thistle

This is the highest rated herb for liver health. The liver is one of the key organs that we focus on with all of our patients, and is responsible for hundreds of functions within the body. Milk thistle has been found to contribute towards the growth of new liver cells. Multiple studies suggest major benefits of taking milk thistle, either through a tincture, a tea or a capsule. In long-term studies, milk thistle was found to improve liver function and decrease the number of deaths in patients with liver disease. Nevertheless, we treat the whole body collectively and in most cases, all organs, including the liver, require attention.

Cleavers

In previous volumes we have discussed the lymphatic system and its importance in cleansing the body's tissue and blood.

Cleavers is a powerful herb that supports the lymphatic system's mechanism. We use this herb with the majority of patients – it is a strong blood purifier, and a reliable diuretic which will help cleanse the urinary tract. It is crucial to stimulate and support the lymphatic system if you are to eliminate acidic waste from your healing body.

Allspice

This fragrant spice acts as a stimulant for the digestive system whilst relaxing any stomach cramping that may be present. We use Allspice quite often during the early detoxification stages. Some patients enjoy sprinkling it over their fruit meals. You are welcome to experiment with this too.

Black Walnut

Eradicating parasites from the gut is one of the keys to overcoming specific "junk food" cravings that are experienced during detoxification. Black walnut is a powerful antifungal herb that is well known for terminating parasites. We rate this herb highly if you are experiencing severe cravings for meat / dairy products during the high fruit detoxification regimen.

Wormwood

As its name suggests, this herb has been used for hundreds of years to expel all variety of worms from the colon and intestinal regions. Cleansing these areas within the body contributes heavily towards correcting any imbalances and removing disease. Wormwood also contains Artemisinin which modern-day science has found to have multiple health benefits. We have found that it significantly impacts on the reversing of autoimmune disorders – with most "diseases" being some form of an autoimmune condition, and stemming from the colon (and digestive tract).

Wild Cherry

A decongestant and a major supporter of the lungs, this herb is used for the upper body blood circulation and serves as a natural treatment for a series of conditions that relate to fevers, pains, coughs and poor digestion.

Blue Vervain

Calming for the central nervous system, Vervain has been used by herbal healers for many centuries. Vervain's healing properties are attributed primarily to its stimulating effect on the liver and other related organs, as well as its relaxing effect on the nervous system. It will bring calmness to nerve tissue whilst decongesting the body's organs. You will experience an overall feeling of wellbeing.

Shepherd's Purse

This herb acts as a detergent and cleanser for the body. It has valuable detoxification properties – it is an anti-diarrheal, anti-mucus, anti-oxidant and anti-inflammatory herb. It is very good for flushing out any stagnant acids in the urinary tract. Several studies highlight that shepherd's purse reduces mucus inflammation, and protects against ulcers, and the slow growth of tumours. Additionally, it will stimulate overall blood circulation and increase the regularity of urination.

Yarrow Flower

Used mainly for the repair and healing of internal organs, this is another highly recommended herb that supports the urinary tract and kidneys with the purpose of filtering out accumulated acidic waste – making provision for the body to heal.

Chickweed

Chickweed relieves minor pain and inflammation whilst acting as a diuretic which reduces fluid retention – this is a common problem with a body that is struggling. Once excess fluids have been flushed out through regular urination, the organs are able to work more effectively (especially the heart).

Black Cumin Seeds

Also known as Nigella Sativa, this herb is one of the longest serving in the history of herbs. It has been used for over 3,300 years, since their first reported discovery in the Egyptian Pharoah Tutankhamun's tomb. Regarded throughout the entire Middle East as one of the most powerful anti-inflammatory herbs, these seeds will support your immune and digestive systems whilst bringing you improved health. There are also religious texts that state the importance of black cumin seed oil, for example, one of the "Hadith" books of Islam states: "there is healing in black seed for all diseases except death". We have found that taken alongside a raw vegan routine, the results could be significant.

Dandelion Root

This herb is well known for its ability to increase bowel movements and urination frequency (diuretic). It will work towards alkalizing your body, and decreasing inflammation and swelling. Many choose to consume it as a tea. As with all herbs mentioned in this book, it is quite a powerful herb and so it should be prescribed with caution to the elderly. Start with small amounts and adjust this based on feel and progression.

Valerian Root

Valerian is most commonly used to help relax an over-active mind at night time and overcome sleep disorders. We also tend to use it for conditions that are related to mental health including psychological stress, depression, anxiety, fear, and for any immediate pains in the upper body region (headaches, migraines).

Liquorice Root

We use this herb with the majority of patients due to its ability to combat stressful events, lift mood, and positively impact the functioning of the kidneys through its support of the adrenal glands. It should be noted that intermittent dry fasting is initially a stressful event for the body and so it is important that we are taking liquorice root during this phase - it will offer great backing to the adrenal glands so they are able to help carry you through these events.

Parsley

A natural detoxifier that gently increases kidney filtration and improves digestion, parsley is used for purifying the blood and it is very effective when used for removing toxic metals from the body. If you have had mercury fillings fitted into your dental cavities, we recommend having these removed and replaced with non-metal fillings (composite, ceramic), and then continue your detoxification with parsley included into the protocol.

Ginkgo Biloba

This herb is a great antioxidant and is used to increase upper body (including the heart) and brain (eyes included) blood circulation. It is very healing and comes with many therapeutic benefits. We recommend this herb highly during regular daily life.

Slippery Elm Bark

We found that the majority of chronically sick patients have a highly congested colon with the walls being plastered as a result of many years of poor eating habits (dairy, starches and meats). We do perform enemas on patients in severe chronic states but in general, we recommend the use of bowel stimulating herbs such as Slippery Elm Bark and Cascara Sagrada. They have been proven to really move all parts of the colon – including the important region of the transverse colon. After taking these herbs, you will start to notice much older, darker and foul-smelling faecal matter leave your body upon each visit to the bathroom - a positive sign that your body is being cleared out.

Cascara Sagrada

This is a very effective herb for cleansing the colon. It comes with a strong laxative effect and will support your detoxification efforts. We tend to prescribe this herb alongside slippery elm bark but it can also be taken alone with positive results.

Hawthorn Berry

This herb has featured in multiple cardiovascular studies and is definitely a powerful blood circulator – specifically focused on heart health. It dilates the blood vessels leading to and from the heart and improves overall blood circulation. Through stimulating bile and gastric secretions, hawthorn berries also strengthen digestion, and this will greatly contribute towards detoxification and healing. We tend to not use this herb with cancer patients or those with tumours (benign or malignant).

Sunshine

Finally, we would like to end with planet earth's natural healing source – the sun. Through our work, we have made a variety of discoveries - one of the key ones being related to vitamin D deficiency. All of our chronic stage patients have had this deficiency in common. The sun truly does heal the human body and so it is important for us to get enough of it on a daily basis. We recognise that in some parts of the world, the sun is not always available so freely. In these cases, we suggest you either move to the nearest sun-dense country (at least for the period it takes to heal), or temporarily take a high quality vitamin D3 supplement. The body will heal much faster with the support of natural sun light. Using the heat from the sun in order to sweat will also add to your health greatly.

We hope that this comprehensive list is helpful to you and your loved ones. We encourage our readers to continue to expand and grow their knowledge. Don't let your reading end here – go on and learn more about these herbs and others that could offer you benefit.

Stay focused – remain persistent – keep learning and expanding your knowledge.

Wishing you all the best. Good luck with your healing journey.

Our Story

It was a Sunday night, over 7 years ago – I was in bed – tossing and turning – unable to sleep. I watched the time pass, from 11pm, to 12am... to 1:30am. I just couldn't sleep. I could feel an immense pressure in my chest cavity and all across my diaphragm area. I couldn't understand where this was coming from. I got up and had some water, I then tried to use the bathroom – the discomfort was still there. Nothing seemed to work – I felt like I was being suffocated each time I would lie down. In the end, I fell asleep out of sheer fatigue.

At the time, I was a sufferer of asthma, eczema, anxiety attacks, and a damaged/leaky gut. These conditions had lead to many symptoms that doctors could not offer me any answers for. I had many tests done but nothing could tell me what the root causes of my problems were.

I started researching about my symptoms, and as I did this, I found myself expanding into the area of medical history. As my research continued, I came to understand that our ancestors lived healthy and long lives, without the health challenges of today.

Eventually, I stumbled upon a few health forums which I joined. Through these, I met a series of individuals that were battling a variety of conditions themselves (a rare genetic disorder, Crohn's disease, multiple sclerosis, muscular dystrophy (MD), diabetes, cushing's disease, a series of 'incurable' autoimmune diseases, and cancer).

We all came together and as we started to grow as a group, we made a significant discovery - that actually the cure to all diseases was discovered back in the 1920s by a Dr Arnold Ehret.

As we studied his material, we started applying his information and protocols on ourselves. This seemed like one experiment worth trying, and within 2 weeks, regardless of our individual conditions, we all started to notice a difference in our improved digestion, higher energy levels, increased mental clarity and improved physical ability. A major change was taking place – our health was improving, as our conditions were decreasing.

We continued to expand our knowledge and we started to encounter even more communities and learnt that there were more magnificent and very gifted healers out there. We came across the works and achievements of Dr Sebi, and completed an insightful and very informative course by Dr Robert Morse.

The essential message of these great healers was very similar to that of Dr Arnold Ehret. Now we had even further confirmation that the information we had been following thus far was in fact THE path to health success. With our progress so far, we could sense victory.

Within 3 months, 30 to 40 percent of our symptoms had disappeared and our health was becoming stronger. Some of us started to take specific herbs in order to enhance the detoxification.

Another 3 months on and the majority of us no longer experienced any more symptoms. Our blood work had also improved significantly, but we still had work to do in order to completely heal.

Now that we had made significant progress in reversing our conditions through self-experimentation, we started to offer basic healthy eating advice to the sick within our local communities.

Eventually, we started working with local patients on a voluntary basis. It was heartbreaking to witness lives being cut short or chronic sickness being accepted as a way of life – all whilst the lifelong eating habits of these individuals remained. The most common diseases that we were coming across included: cancers, heart disease, chronic kidney disease, high blood pressure, varying infections, and diabetes.

By helping our communities with changing their daily eating habits, we started seeing results, and although the transitional phase of moving from the foods that they were so used to eating, to moving over to a raw plant-based routine was a challenge, in the end, it was worth the shift. Note: there were many that ignored our advice and sadly they continued to remain in their state.

We did have resistance initially from family members and friends of the sick but after some time as they started seeing health improvements, more started joining us, and they also started experiencing what we had when we first set out on our journey of natural self-healing.

Nevertheless, challenges still remained – the main ones being the undoing of society's programming that cooked food is an essential part of life (including animal and wheat based products) and raw food alone surely cannot be good for you. It doesn't take long to explain how to remove imbalances and dis-ease from within the human body but the more extensive task is to actually have the protocol information applied and adhered to completely.

This is where the idea for this series of journal & progress tracker stemmed from. We felt compelled to spread this information in a more digestible and applicable form, over a series of volumes, in which we would start by offering some key informative points, followed by a journal which would allow for you to actually apply the information, record your progress, daily feelings and stay accountable to yourself. We also found that journaling and writing to oneself really helps to self-motivate and enhances a self consciousness that is needed when following a protocol like this.

Each journal volume within this series will be designed to help you record your journey for a 30 day period. At the start of each journal we will continue to offer insightful information about our experiences, whilst expanding on and re-iterating specific parts of this protocol.

The fact that you are reading this foreword is an indication that you are already on your way to self-healing. Regardless of your condition, we invite you to seek more knowledge and set your health free.

May you always remain blessed and guided.

Much Love From The Health Central Team

Important Notes for Overcoming Your Catatonia

1. It should be noted that based on our experiences and understanding, whether your condition is Catatonia, or any other, we recommend the same raw vegan healing protocol across all spectrums. With some conditions, you may need to perform a deeper detoxification (using herbs - or organ/glandular meat/capsules for more chronic situations) before achieving significant results, but in general, we have found this protocol to work in most cases. In our experience, the goal is not to cure, but instead to raise health levels first, through healthy food choices, as intended for our species – before the eradication and prevention of these modern-day "disease" conditions can take place.

2. With all conditions, we have found that the lymphatic system has become congested and overwhelmed due to the kidneys not efficiently filtering out the accumulated cell waste – as a result of years of dehydrating cooked/wheat/dairy foods. The adrenal glands work closely with the kidneys, and so adrenal/kidney herbs and glandular formulas played a major role in opening up these channels. We also found that opening up the bowels and loosening the gut was hugely important too.

3. The healing protocol that we used on ourselves is discussed and expanded upon throughout the various volumes in this series. Our goal is to share information that we have gathered from our journeys, and let you decide if it is something that you feel could also work for you in your

journey for health and vitality. You are not obliged to use this information, and you may proceed as you see fit.

Through our study, research and application, we have found this system to correct any internal imbalances and remove dis-ease that has occurred within the human body, due to the continued consumption of acid-forming foods.

4. Always take progression ultra slow and go at your own pace. Listen to your body at every stage. We cannot re-iterate this point enough. Pay attention to how you feel and continue to consult your doctor and monitor your blood work.

5. A special emphasis needs to be given to the transition phase when moving from your regular, standard diet, to a raw vegan diet that is high in fruit. You must take your time and slowly remove foods from your current routine, and replace them with either fasting or a small amount of fruit in the initial stages. Work with small amounts – please do not make any drastic changes. If you do not feel comfortable or have any concerns at any stage, please immediately stop.

Note: with any dietary change, this can be a stressful event for the body and so it is important that you support your kidneys and adrenal glands using the appropriate herbs and glandular formulas previously mentioned.

6. Before partaking in any new dietary routine, please always consult your Doctor first and ensure that they are aware of your health related goals. This approach is beneficial because (a) you can monitor your blood work with your doctor as you progress with this new protocol, and (b) if you are on any medication, as your health improves, you

can review its need and/or discuss having dosage amounts reduced (if necessary).

7. Please note that we are sharing information from our collective experiences of how we healed ourselves from a variety of diseases and conditions. These are solely our own opinions. Having reversed a range of conditions using essentially the same protocol, our understanding and conclusion, based on our experience alone, is that regardless of the disease, illness or condition name – removing it from the human body stems from correcting your diet and transitioning over to a more raw vegan lifestyle.

8. Proceed with care, and again, do not make any sudden changes – always take your time in slowly removing foods that are not serving you, and replacing them with high energy sweet tree-ripened juicy fruit. If at any point you feel that you are moving too quickly, please adjust your transition accordingly. Results may vary between individuals.

9. We recommended that you constantly expand your knowledge and familiarise yourself with the works of Dr Arnold Ehret, Dr Robert Morse and John Rose. When you feel confident with your understanding, start taking gradual steps towards reaching your goals. Make the most of this journal and use it to serve you as a companion on your journey.

The Power of Journaling

a) Journaling your inner self talk is a truly effective way of increasing self awareness and consciousness. To be able to transfer your thoughts and feelings onto a piece of paper is a truly effective method of self reflection and improvement. This is much needed when you are switching to a high fruit dietary routine.

b) Be sure to always add the date of journaling at the top of each page used. This is invaluable for when you wish to go back and review/track progress and your feelings/thoughts on previous dates.

c) Keep a comprehensive record of activities, thoughts, and really log everything you ate/are eating. You can even make miscellaneous notes if you feel that they will help you.

d) We have added tips and questions to offer you guidance, reminders, inspiration and areas to journal about.

e) We like to use journals to have a conversation with ourselves. Inner talk can really help you overcome any challenges that you are experiencing. Express yourself and any concerns that you may have.

f) Try to advise yourself as though you are your best friend – similarly to how you would advise a close friend or family member. You will be surprised at the results that you will achieve from using this technique.

g) Add notes to this journal and work your way through the 30 days. Once completed, move onto the next journal volume in this series, which will also be structured in a similar, supportive and educational fashion. We have produced a series of these journals in order to cater for your ongoing journey and goals.

h) For those of you who would like to track your progress with a more basic notebook-style journal, we have produced a separate series in which each notebook interior differs. This is to cater for your complete health journaling needs.

We have laid out the following examples to serve as potential frameworks for one way of how a journal could be filled in on a daily basis. These are just basic examples, but you can complete your daily journals in any other way that you feel is most comfortable and effective for you.

[EXAMPLE 1]
[EXAMPLE 1]
Today's Date: 3rd Jan 2020

Morning
Dry fasting (water and food free since 8pm last night) - will go up until 12:30pm today, and start with 500ml of spring water before eating half a watermelon.

Afternoon
Kept busy and was in and out quite a bit - so nothing consumed.

Evening
At around 5pm, I had a peppermint tea with a selection of mixed dried fruit (small bowl of apricot, dates, mango, pineapple, and prunes).

Night
Sipped on spring water through the evening as required.
Finished off the other half of the watermelon from the morning.

Today's Notes (Highlights, Thoughts, Feelings):

As with most days, today started well with me dry fasting (continuing my fast from my sleep/skipping breakfast) up until around 12:30pm and then eating half a watermelon. The laxative effect of the watermelon helped me poop and release any loosened toxins from the fasting period.
I tend to struggle on some days from 3pm onwards. Up until that point I am okay but if the cravings strike then it can be challenging. I remind myself that those burgers and chips do not have any live healing energy.
I feel good in general. I feel fantastic doing a fruit/juice fast but slightly empty by the end of the day.
Cooked food makes me feel severe fatigue and mental fog.
Will continue with my fruit fasting and start to introduce fruit juices due to their deeper detox benefits. I would love to be on juices only as I have seen others within the community achieve amazing results.

[EXAMPLE 2]
Today's Date: 4th Jan 2020

Morning

Today I woke and my children were enjoying some watermelon for breakfast – and the smell was luring so I joined them. Large bowl of watermelon eaten at around 8am. Started with a glass of water.

Afternoon

Snacked on left over watermelon throughout the morning and afternoon. Had 5 dates an hour or so after.

Evening

Had around 3 mangoes at around 6pm. Felt content – but then I was invited round to a family gathering where a selection of pizzas, burgers and chips were being served. I gave into the peer pressure and felt like I let myself down!

Night

Having over-eaten earlier on in the evening, I was still feeling bloated with a headache (possibly digestion related) and I also felt quite mucus filled (wheez in chest and coughing up phlegm). Very sleepy and low energy. The perils of cooked foods!!

Today's Notes (Highlights, Thoughts, Feelings):

I let myself down today. It all started well until I ate a fully blown meal (and over-ate). I didn't remain focussed and I spun off track. As a result my energy levels were much lower and I felt a bout of extreme fatigue 30 minutes after the meal (most likely the body struggling to with digesting all that cooked food).
I need to stick to the plan because the difference between fruit fasting, and eating cooked foods is huge – 1 makes you feel empowered whilst the other makes you feel drained. I also felt the mucus overload after the meal – it kicked in pretty quickly.
Today I felt disappointed after giving in to the meal but tomorrow is a new day and I will keep on going! It is important to remind myself that I won't get better if I cannot stick to the routine.

1. Today's Date:

—————————— Morning ——————————
(work towards continuing your night time dry fast up until at least 12pm)

—————————— Afternoon ——————————
(get hydrating with fresh fruit or even better slow juiced fruits/berries/melons)

—————————— Evening ——————————
(aim to wind down to a dry fast by around 6pm to 7pm)

—————————— Night ——————————
(work your way up to dry fasting from the evening until 12pm the following day)

Today's Notes (Highlights, Thoughts, Feelings, What Could You Improve On?)

"Get yourself an accountability partner to complete a 30 day detox with. Start with 7 days and work your way up. It will be fun and motivating completing it with somebody (or a group) ...or of course you can go it alone."

2. Today's Date:

Morning
(work towards continuing your night time dry fast up until at least 12pm)

Afternoon
(get hydrating with fresh fruit or even better slow juiced fruits/berries/melons)

Evening
(aim to wind down to a dry fast by around 6pm to 7pm)

Night
(work your way up to dry fasting from the evening until 12pm the following day)

Today's Notes (Highlights, Thoughts, Feelings, What Could You Improve On?)

"Remember when starting out, it is important to keep yourself hydrated throughout the day. Spring Water is a good start - and slow/cold pressed juice is also very powerful."

3. Today's Date:

—————————————— **Morning** ——————————————

(work towards continuing your night time dry fast up until at least 12pm)

—————————————— **Afternoon** ——————————————

(get hydrating with fresh fruit or even better slow juiced fruits/berries/melons)

—————————————— **Evening** ——————————————

(aim to wind down to a dry fast by around 6pm to 7pm)

—————————————— **Night** ——————————————

(work your way up to dry fasting from the evening until 12pm the following day)

Today's Notes (Highlights, Thoughts, Feelings, What Could You Improve On?)

"Eat melons/watermelons separately, and before any other fruit as it digests faster and we want to limit fermentation (acidity) which can occur if other fruits are mixed in."

4. Today's Date:

Morning
(work towards continuing your night time dry fast up until at least 12pm)

Afternoon
(get hydrating with fresh fruit or even better slow juiced fruits/berries/melons)

Evening
(aim to wind down to a dry fast by around 6pm to 7pm)

Night
(work your way up to dry fasting from the evening until 12pm the following day)

Today's Notes (Highlights, Thoughts, Feelings, What Could You Improve On?)

"Stay focussed on the end goal of removing mucus & toxins from your body and feeling wonderful! Look forward to being full of vitality and disease free once again"

5. Today's Date:

Morning
(work towards continuing your night time dry fast up until at least 12pm)

Afternoon
(get hydrating with fresh fruit or even better slow juiced fruits/berries/melons)

Evening
(aim to wind down to a dry fast by around 6pm to 7pm)

Night
(work your way up to dry fasting from the evening until 12pm the following day)

Today's Notes (Highlights, Thoughts, Feelings, What Could You Improve On?)

"Meditate and perform deep breathing exercises in order to help yourself remain present minded and on track. Perform these techniques throughout the day but also during any challenging times that you may come to face."

6. Today's Date:

Morning
(work towards continuing your night time dry fast up until at least 12pm)

Afternoon
(get hydrating with fresh fruit or even better slow juiced fruits/berries/melons)

Evening
(aim to wind down to a dry fast by around 6pm to 7pm)

Night
(work your way up to dry fasting from the evening until 12pm the following day)

Today's Notes (Highlights, Thoughts, Feelings, What Could You Improve On?)

"Join a few like-minded communities – there are many juicing and raw vegan based groups, both online and offline. Being part of a community can help motivate you to reach your goals. You will also learn a great amount from others. Seeing others succeed is empowering."

7. Today's Date:

Morning
(work towards continuing your night time dry fast up until at least 12pm)

Afternoon
(get hydrating with fresh fruit or even better slow juiced fruits/berries/melons)

Evening
(aim to wind down to a dry fast by around 6pm to 7pm)

Night
(work your way up to dry fasting from the evening until 12pm the following day)

Today's Notes (Highlights, Thoughts, Feelings, What Could You Improve On?)

"If you are struggling to cope with hunger
pangs in the early stages, try some dates
or dried apricots, prunes, or raisins, with
a cup of herbal tea. However, these pangs will disappear
once your body adjusts to your new routine."

8. Today's Date:

Morning
(work towards continuing your night time dry fast up until at least 12pm)

Afternoon
(get hydrating with fresh fruit or even better slow juiced fruits/berries/melons)

Evening
(aim to wind down to a dry fast by around 6pm to 7pm)

Night
(work your way up to dry fasting from the evening until 12pm the following day)

Today's Notes (Highlights, Thoughts, Feelings, What Could You Improve On?)

"Get into a routine of regularly buying fresh fruit (or grow your own if weather permits) to keep your supplies up. Local wholesale markets do also clear fruits/veg on Fridays (if they are closed for the weekend) at a lower price, so they are worth a visit."

9. Today's Date:

Morning

(work towards continuing your night time dry fast up until at least 12pm)

Afternoon

(get hydrating with fresh fruit or even better slow juiced fruits/berries/melons)

Evening

(aim to wind down to a dry fast by around 6pm to 7pm)

Night

(work your way up to dry fasting from the evening until 12pm the following day)

Today's Notes (Highlights, Thoughts, Feelings, What Could You Improve On?)

"Regularly remind yourself about the great rewards and benefits that you will experience by keeping up this detoxification process. Imagine the lives you could save as a result of healing yourself."

10. Today's Date:

Morning
(work towards continuing your night time dry fast up until at least 12pm)

Afternoon
(get hydrating with fresh fruit or even better slow juiced fruits/berries/melons)

Evening
(aim to wind down to a dry fast by around 6pm to 7pm)

Night
(work your way up to dry fasting from the evening until 12pm the following day)

Today's Notes (Highlights, Thoughts, Feelings, What Could You Improve On?)

"Keep your teeth brushed (using miswak; a natural brush). Use coconut oil to oil pull before bedtime. Done correctly, you will notice an improvement in your dental health with these practices."

11. Today's Date:

Morning
(work towards continuing your night time dry fast up until at least 12pm)

Afternoon
(get hydrating with fresh fruit or even better slow juiced fruits/berries/melons)

Evening
(aim to wind down to a dry fast by around 6pm to 7pm)

Night
(work your way up to dry fasting from the evening until 12pm the following day)

Today's Notes (Highlights, Thoughts, Feelings, What Could You Improve On?)

"Be motivated by the vision of becoming an example for others to learn from and follow. You could change the lives of family and friends by showing them your own improvements."

12. Today's Date:

Morning
(work towards continuing your night time dry fast up until at least 12pm)

Afternoon
(get hydrating with fresh fruit or even better slow juiced fruits/berries/melons)

Evening
(aim to wind down to a dry fast by around 6pm to 7pm)

Night
(work your way up to dry fasting from the evening until 12pm the following day)

Today's Notes (Highlights, Thoughts, Feelings, What Could You Improve On?)

"Embrace your achievements and wonderful results – feel and appreciate the difference within you as a result of this new routine. Notice how your personal agility and fitness has improved. Feel the improved energy levels."

13. Today's Date:

Morning
(work towards continuing your night time dry fast up until at least 12pm)

Afternoon
(get hydrating with fresh fruit or even better slow juiced fruits/berries/melons)

Evening
(aim to wind down to a dry fast by around 6pm to 7pm)

Night
(work your way up to dry fasting from the evening until 12pm the following day)

Today's Notes (Highlights, Thoughts, Feelings, What Could You Improve On?)

"Buy fruit in bulk where possible so you have ample supplies for a week or two in advance. If in a hot climate, you could even freeze your fruit or make ice lollies out of it (crush & freeze). Immerse yourself in fruit so it becomes your only option."

14. Today's Date:

Morning
(work towards continuing your night time dry fast up until at least 12pm)

Afternoon
(get hydrating with fresh fruit or even better slow juiced fruits/berries/melons)

Evening
(aim to wind down to a dry fast by around 6pm to 7pm)

Night
(work your way up to dry fasting from the evening until 12pm the following day)

Today's Notes (Highlights, Thoughts, Feelings, What Could You Improve On?)

"Stay as busy as you can during the daytime. Creating a busy routine makes it easier to manage your diet. Have a purpose, and keep setting yourself new tasks/actions in order to keep yourself occupied."

15. Today's Date:

Morning
(work towards continuing your night time dry fast up until at least 12pm)

Afternoon
(get hydrating with fresh fruit or even better slow juiced fruits/berries/melons)

Evening
(aim to wind down to a dry fast by around 6pm to 7pm)

Night
(work your way up to dry fasting from the evening until 12pm the following day)

Today's Notes (Highlights, Thoughts, Feelings, What Could You Improve On?)

"Complete your fruit and fasting routine with a group of friends/family/colleagues so you can all support one another. Make it fun - set challenges - dry fast together and break your fasts together - have weekly catch up sessions."

16. Today's Date:

Morning
(work towards continuing your night time dry fast up until at least 12pm)

Afternoon
(get hydrating with fresh fruit or even better slow juiced fruits/berries/melons)

Evening
(aim to wind down to a dry fast by around 6pm to 7pm)

Night
(work your way up to dry fasting from the evening until 12pm the following day)

Today's Notes (Highlights, Thoughts, Feelings, What Could You Improve On?)

"Look out for white cloud/sediment (acids) in your urine to confirm that your kidneys are filtering out waste. Urinate in a glass jar - leave for 2 hours to settle before observing."

17. Today's Date:

Morning
(work towards continuing your night time dry fast up until at least 12pm)

Afternoon
(get hydrating with fresh fruit or even better slow juiced fruits/berries/melons)

Evening
(aim to wind down to a dry fast by around 6pm to 7pm)

Night
(work your way up to dry fasting from the evening until 12pm the following day)

Today's Notes (Highlights, Thoughts, Feelings, What Could You Improve On?)

"Have genuine love and care for yourself. If you are craving junk food, affirm positive inner talk ("I won't feel good after eating junk. I love myself too much to put my body through that - so leave it out!"). You can also take Sea Kelp, Coconut Water, or Celery to reduce any salt cravings."

18. Today's Date:

Morning
(work towards continuing your night time dry fast up until at least 12pm)

Afternoon
(get hydrating with fresh fruit or even better slow juiced fruits/berries/melons)

Evening
(aim to wind down to a dry fast by around 6pm to 7pm)

Night
(work your way up to dry fasting from the evening until 12pm the following day)

Today's Notes (Highlights, Thoughts, Feelings, What Could You Improve On?)

"Feel and note down the difference within yourself as you filter out unwanted acids with this alkaline, water-dense high fruit protocol."

19. Today's Date:

Morning
(work towards continuing your night time dry fast up until at least 12pm)

Afternoon
(get hydrating with fresh fruit or even better slow juiced fruits/berries/melons)

Evening
(aim to wind down to a dry fast by around 6pm to 7pm)

Night
(work your way up to dry fasting from the evening until 12pm the following day)

Today's Notes (Highlights, Thoughts, Feelings, What Could You Improve On?)

"Look for acidic waste/sediments in your urine regularly in order to ensure your kidneys are filtering. Dry fasting for over 18 hours will increase kidney filtration. You can also drink the juice of slow-juiced citrus fruits (lemons, oranges). Sweating helps too."

20. Today's Date:

Morning

(work towards continuing your night time dry fast up until at least 12pm)

Afternoon

(get hydrating with fresh fruit or even better slow juiced fruits/berries/melons)

Evening

(aim to wind down to a dry fast by around 6pm to 7pm)

Night

(work your way up to dry fasting from the evening until 12pm the following day)

Today's Notes (Highlights, Thoughts, Feelings, What Could You Improve On?)

"Infections emerge in an acidic environment. In order
to remove infections, you must concentrate on kidney
filtration. Use herbs for kidneys and adrenal glands - using
dry fasting to assist."

21. Today's Date:

—— Morning ——
(work towards continuing your night time dry fast up until at least 12pm)

—— Afternoon ——
(get hydrating with fresh fruit or even better slow juiced fruits/berries/melons)

—— Evening ——
(aim to wind down to a dry fast by around 6pm to 7pm)

—— Night ——
(work your way up to dry fasting from the evening until 12pm the following day)

Today's Notes (Highlights, Thoughts, Feelings, What Could You Improve On?)

"Any deficiencies that you may have will start to disappear once you have cleansed your congested gut/colon, kidneys and various other eliminative organs."

22. Today's Date:

Morning
(work towards continuing your night time dry fast up until at least 12pm)

Afternoon
(get hydrating with fresh fruit or even better slow juiced fruits/berries/melons)

Evening
(aim to wind down to a dry fast by around 6pm to 7pm)

Night
(work your way up to dry fasting from the evening until 12pm the following day)

Today's Notes (Highlights, Thoughts, Feelings, What Could You Improve On?)

"Dependant on how deeply you detoxify yourself, it is possible to eliminate any genetic weaknesses that you may have inherited. This will require a deep detoxification process which involves juicing your fruits with prolonged periods of dry fasting"

23. Today's Date:

Morning

(work towards continuing your night time dry fast up until at least 12pm)

Afternoon

(get hydrating with fresh fruit or even better slow juiced fruits/berries/melons)

Evening

(aim to wind down to a dry fast by around 6pm to 7pm)

Night

(work your way up to dry fasting from the evening until 12pm the following day)

Today's Notes (Highlights, Thoughts, Feelings, What Could You Improve On?)

"Stay focused on your detoxification for deeper, lasting results. All past injuries / trauma are also repairable for good. Get those old acids out and replace them with a pain-free alkaline environment"

24. Today's Date:

Morning
(work towards continuing your night time dry fast up until at least 12pm)

Afternoon
(get hydrating with fresh fruit or even better slow juiced fruits/berries/melons)

Evening
(aim to wind down to a dry fast by around 6pm to 7pm)

Night
(work your way up to dry fasting from the evening until 12pm the following day)

Today's Notes (Highlights, Thoughts, Feelings, What Could You Improve On?)

"If you suffer from ongoing sadness / depression, a deep detox will support your mental health. You will soon notice a positive change in your mood. **Note:** *you will need to support your adrenal glands and kidneys with glandulars and/or herbs (liqorice root, sea kelp, uva ursi, nettle)"*

25. Today's Date:

Morning
(work towards continuing your night time dry fast up until at least 12pm)

Afternoon
(get hydrating with fresh fruit or even better slow juiced fruits/berries/melons)

Evening
(aim to wind down to a dry fast by around 6pm to 7pm)

Night
(work your way up to dry fasting from the evening until 12pm the following day)

Today's Notes (Highlights, Thoughts, Feelings, What Could You Improve On?)

"Have your fruits/ juices throughout the day - with dry fasting gaps of at least 3 hours in-between each feed. As the evening approaches, start to dry fast fully – from this point on, your body wants to rest and heal."

26. Today's Date:

Morning
(work towards continuing your night time dry fast up until at least 12pm)

Afternoon
(get hydrating with fresh fruit or even better slow juiced fruits/berries/melons)

Evening
(aim to wind down to a dry fast by around 6pm to 7pm)

Night
(work your way up to dry fasting from the evening until 12pm the following day)

Today's Notes (Highlights, Thoughts, Feelings, What Could You Improve On?)

"The kidneys dislike proteins but really appreciate juicy fruits like melons, berries, citrus fruits, pineapples, mangoes, apples, grapes. Witness the difference by replacing cooked foods and protein with fruits. Become the change."

27. Today's Date:

Morning
(work towards continuing your night time dry fast up until at least 12pm)

Afternoon
(get hydrating with fresh fruit or even better slow juiced fruits/berries/melons)

Evening
(aim to wind down to a dry fast by around 6pm to 7pm)

Night
(work your way up to dry fasting from the evening until 12pm the following day)

Today's Notes (Highlights, Thoughts, Feelings, What Could You Improve On?)

"Healing is very easy. There's no need to complicate it. Keep everything simple and you will see results. Concentrate on improving your level of health to a point where dis-ease is dissolved"

28. Today's Date:

Morning
(work towards continuing your night time dry fast up until at least 12pm)

Afternoon
(get hydrating with fresh fruit or even better slow juiced fruits/berries/melons)

Evening
(aim to wind down to a dry fast by around 6pm to 7pm)

Night
(work your way up to dry fasting from the evening until 12pm the following day)

Today's Notes (Highlights, Thoughts, Feelings, What Could You Improve On?)

"Keep your body in an alkaline and hydrated state as this is where regeneration takes place - and disease cannot continue to exist. You can achieve this through a raw fruits and vegetables diet (find your balance between the two)"

29. Today's Date:

Morning
(work towards continuing your night time dry fast up until at least 12pm)

Afternoon
(get hydrating with fresh fruit or even better slow juiced fruits/berries/melons)

Evening
(aim to wind down to a dry fast by around 6pm to 7pm)

Night
(work your way up to dry fasting from the evening until 12pm the following day)

Today's Notes (Highlights, Thoughts, Feelings, What Could You Improve On?)

"An enema with boiled water (cooled down) can support your detox. However this high fruit dietary protocol will encourage healthy bowel movement and this should be sufficient, unless if you are at a chronic stage."

30. Today's Date:

Morning
(work towards continuing your night time dry fast up until at least 12pm)

Afternoon
(get hydrating with fresh fruit or even better slow juiced fruits/berries/melons)

Evening
(aim to wind down to a dry fast by around 6pm to 7pm)

Night
(work your way up to dry fasting from the evening until 12pm the following day)

Today's Notes (Highlights, Thoughts, Feelings, What Could You Improve On?)

"You can have your iris' read by an iridologist that works with Dr Bernard Jensen's system. An Iris Diagnosis will offer you information on specific areas of weakness that pre-exist for you to focus on."

Made in the USA
Monee, IL
13 January 2024

51742177R00048